GESTATIONAL DIABETES COOKBOOK

TABLE OF CONTENT

INTRODUCTION

Gestational diabetes, a temporary yet impactful condition, emerges during pregnancy and necessitates a vigilant approach to dietary choices for the health and well-being of both the expectant mother and her developing child. This unique form of diabetes occurs when the body cannot produce or utilize insulin effectively to manage increased blood sugar levels during pregnancy. Unlike pre-existing types of diabetes, gestational diabetes typically manifests around the 24th to 28th week of pregnancy and often subsides after childbirth. However, its potential consequences are far-reaching and require meticulous attention, particularly in the realm of diet. The food choices made during this critical time can play a pivotal role in managing blood sugar levels, safeguarding the health of the baby, and mitigating risks for both the mother and child. This book delves into the intricate relationship between gestational diabetes and diet, shedding light on the principles, strategies, and dietary considerations that can help expectant mothers navigate this temporary but significant health challenge with confidence and care. We will start a journey through the nutritional landscape of gestational diabetes, exploring not only what to eat but also why, how, and when, all aimed at fostering a healthy pregnancy and ensuring a bright and flourishing future for both mother and child.

UNDERSTANDING GESTATIONAL DIABETES

Understanding gestational diabetes is paramount for expectant mothers and healthcare providers alike, as this condition poses unique challenges during pregnancy. Gestational diabetes is a temporary form of diabetes that typically develops in the second or third trimester, affecting around 2-10% of pregnant women. It arises when the body cannot produce or use insulin efficiently to control blood sugar levels, resulting in elevated glucose in the bloodstream. While the exact cause remains uncertain, hormonal changes during pregnancy are believed to play a pivotal role in insulin resistance. The implications of gestational diabetes are far-reaching, impacting not only the mother but also the developing fetus. High blood sugar levels can lead to complications such as macrosomia (excessive fetal growth), preeclampsia, and preterm birth. Moreover, babies born to mothers with uncontrolled gestational diabetes may face a higher risk of obesity and type 2 diabetes later in life. Fortunately, with proper management and vigilant monitoring of blood glucose levels, the risks associated with gestational diabetes can be significantly reduced. Lifestyle modifications, including a well-balanced diet, regular physical activity, and in some cases, medication, are often prescribed to keep blood sugar levels in check. Regular prenatal care is essential to monitor the condition's progression and ensure the well-being of both mother and baby. By gaining a comprehensive understanding of gestational diabetes, expectant mothers can take proactive steps to manage their health, reduce potential complications, and ultimately, enjoy a healthier pregnancy journey while safeguarding their child's future well-being. Eating the right thing, having the right diets can go all the way for both you and your child/children

IMPORTANCE OF GESTATIONAL DIET

The importance of a gestational diet cannot be overstated, as it plays a fundamental role in the health and well-being of both the expectant mother and her developing baby. A balanced and nutrient-rich gestational diet provides the essential vitamins, minerals, and macronutrients necessary for the formation of vital organs, bones, and tissues in the developing fetus. Adequate intake of key nutrients like folic acid, iron, calcium, and protein is crucial to prevent birth defects, support the expansion of the maternal blood volume, and ensure proper bone development in the baby. Additionally, a well-rounded diet can help manage common pregnancy-related discomforts such as nausea, constipation, and fatigue. Furthermore, it contributes to maintaining a healthy weight and blood sugar levels, reducing the risk of gestational diabetes and complications during childbirth. The gestational diet also impacts the mother's long-term health, influencing her post-pregnancy recovery, lactation, and the future health of her child. Therefore, a conscientiously planned and monitored gestational diet is an indispensable component of a healthy pregnancy, promoting optimal growth and setting the stage for a bright and healthy future for both mother and baby.

FOLLOWING A HEALTHY EATING PLAN TO NOURISH YOU AND YOUR BABY

Following a healthy eating plan during pregnancy is paramount to nourishing both you and your growing baby. It's a time when the significance of nutrition takes center stage, as the food choices you make directly impact your baby's development and your own well-being. A balanced diet during pregnancy should encompass a variety of nutrient-rich foods, including fruits, vegetables, whole grains, lean proteins, and dairy products. These foods provide essential vitamins and minerals such as folic acid, calcium, iron, and protein, all of which play pivotal roles in fetal growth, brain development, and overall maternal health. Equally crucial is maintaining proper hydration. Staying well-hydrated aids in digestion, circulation, and the formation of amniotic fluid. Moreover, it's vital to monitor and control your intake of certain foods that may pose risks during pregnancy, such as high-mercury fish and unpasteurized dairy products. Working closely with your healthcare provider or a registered dietitian can help you tailor your eating plan to meet your individual needs and address any specific concerns or dietary restrictions. By prioritizing a nutritious diet throughout your pregnancy journey, you'll be providing your baby with the best possible start in life and supporting your own health and vitality along the way.

SMOOTHIE AND BREAKFASTS

Navigating the dietary landscape during pregnancy can be both exhilarating and challenging, and when gestational diabetes enters the equation, a well-thought-out nutritional strategy becomes paramount. Smoothies and Breakfasts for Gestational Diabetes Diet, helps to empower expectant mothers with delicious, nourishing, and blood sugar-friendly options to kickstart their day. Breakfast, often deemed the most important meal, takes on new significance when managing gestational diabetes. It sets the tone for your blood sugar levels and energy throughout the day. Within these pages, you'll discover a treasure trove of morning delights, from wholesome smoothies brimming with essential nutrients to hearty breakfast recipes tailored to keep blood sugar fluctuations at bay. We aim to make your breakfast choices not only diabetes-friendly but also a delightful and satisfying part of your pregnancy journey.

PEACH VEGGIE SMOOTHIE

The Peach Veggie Smoothie is a delightful fusion of sweet and nutritious, offering a burst of flavor and health BENEFITS in a single glass. This vibrant concoction seamlessly blends the sweetness of ripe peaches with the goodness of nutrient-packed vegetables, resulting in a refreshing and energy-boosting drink that's perfect for breakfast or as a wholesome snack.

BENEFITS

This Peach Veggie Smoothie is a nutritional powerhouse, packing a multitude of BENEFITS for your well-being. Peaches provide a natural sweetness along with vitamins A and C, while the addition of vegetables such as spinach or kale introduces a rich source of fiber, antioxidants, and essential minerals like potassium. This combination not only supports digestive health but also boosts your immune system, aids in managing blood pressure, and promotes radiant skin. Additionally, the fiber content helps regulate blood sugar levels, making it an excellent choice for individuals with diabetes.

PREPARATION

Creating this invigorating Peach Veggie Smoothie is a breeze. Begin by gathering your ingredients, which typically include ripe peaches, a handful of fresh spinach or kale, Greek yogurt or a dairy-free alternative for creaminess, a splash of almond milk, and a touch of honey or a natural sweetener if desired. Simply blend these components until smooth, adjusting the thickness with more or less almond milk to suit your preference. The result is a velvety, peachy-green elixir that can be enjoyed immediately. Feel free to customize your Peach Veggie Smoothie by adding a scoop of protein powder, flaxseeds, or chia seeds for an extra boost of nutrition and satiety.

BERRY AVOCADO SMOOTHIE

The Berry Avocado Smoothie is a vibrant and wholesome delight that encapsulates the essence of health and flavor in a single glass. This delectable concoction combines the irresistible sweetness of mixed berries with the creamy richness of avocado, creating a refreshing and nutritious beverage that not only tantalizes the taste buds but also offers a plethora of health BENEFITS.

BENEFITS

This smoothie is a nutritional powerhouse. The inclusion of berries, such as strawberries, blueberries, and raspberries, infuses it with a burst of antioxidants, vitamins, and fiber, all of which support overall well-being. Avocado, on the other hand, contributes heart-healthy monounsaturated fats, additional fiber, and essential nutrients like potassium and folate. Together, these ingredients provide sustained energy, aid in digestion, promote healthy skin, and may even assist in managing blood sugar levels. Furthermore, the smoothie is an excellent choice for those seeking a filling and satisfying snack or breakfast option that helps control appetite throughout the day.

PREPARATION

Creating this Berry Avocado Smoothie is a breeze. Simply combine a ripe avocado, a cup of mixed berries (fresh or frozen), a banana for natural sweetness, a cup of low-fat yogurt or almond milk for creaminess, and a drizzle of honey or a handful of spinach leaves for an extra nutritional boost. Blend everything together until smooth, and in a matter of minutes, you'll have a refreshing and nutrient-dense beverage ready to kickstart your day or provide a delightful snack. Enjoy the vibrant colors and flavors of this smoothie while nourishing your body with the goodness it deserves.

BANANA CHOCOLATE CHIP BAKED OATMEAL

Banana Chocolate Chip Baked Oatmeal, a delightful fusion of wholesome ingredients, is a breakfast indulgence that offers a balance of taste and nutrition. This dish not only tantalizes your taste buds but also provides a hearty start to your day, making it a perfect choice for those seeking a healthy and delicious breakfast option.

BENEFITS

This scrumptious baked oatmeal packs a nutritional punch. It's rich in dietary fiber, which aids in digestion and helps regulate blood sugar levels – a particularly important factor for individuals with diabetes. Bananas contribute essential vitamins and potassium, promoting heart health and muscle function. Dark chocolate chips add a touch of sweetness without overwhelming your taste buds, and they are known for their antioxidant properties. Moreover, this dish is a source of sustained energy, keeping you satiated throughout the morning.

PREPARATION

Creating Banana Chocolate Chip Baked Oatmeal is a breeze. Start by mashing ripe bananas and mixing them with oats, milk (or a dairy-free alternative), eggs (or egg substitute for a vegan version), a hint of vanilla extract, a touch of sweetener, and a generous sprinkle of dark chocolate chips. After combining the ingredients, pour the mixture into a baking dish and pop it in the oven until it's golden brown and set. The result is a warm, comforting, and nutrient-packed breakfast that's perfect for a leisurely morning or meal prep for busy days. Customize it with nuts or seeds for added texture and nutrition, and enjoy the convenience of having a delicious and healthy breakfast ready to go.

GREEK YOGHURT PARFAIT

In the realm of breakfast options that effortlessly combine health and indulgence, the Greek Yogurt Parfait stands as a shining example. This delightful creation offers a symphony of flavors and textures, while its nutrient-rich composition makes it a stellar choice for those seeking a wholesome start to their day.

BENEFITS

Greek Yogurt Parfait is a nutritional powerhouse, boasting BENEFITS that span beyond its delicious taste. It is a fantastic source of high-quality protein, which helps with satiety and muscle maintenance. Probiotics found in yogurt contribute to gut health and digestion. Additionally, this parfait is laden with vitamins, minerals, and antioxidants from the fruits and nuts used, supporting overall well-being.

PREPARATION

Creating a Greek Yogurt Parfait is a simple yet customizable process. Start with a base of creamy Greek yogurt, renowned for its rich, velvety texture and high protein content. Layer it with fresh, seasonal fruits like berries, sliced bananas, or diced mangoes for a burst of natural sweetness and vitamins. Add a sprinkle of crunchy granola or chopped nuts for texture and healthy fats. Drizzle with honey or maple syrup for a touch of sweetness, if desired. Repeat the layers to create a visually appealing parfait. Serve it in a glass or bowl and savor a balanced, nutrient-packed breakfast that's ready in minutes.

MUSH ROOM THYME FRITTATA

Introducing the Mushroom Thyme Frittata—a culinary masterpiece that not only tantalizes your taste buds but also offers a plethora of health BENEFITS. This savory delight combines the earthy richness of mushrooms with the aromatic essence of thyme, resulting in a wholesome dish that's perfect for any meal of the day.

BENEFITS

Beyond its delectable taste, the Mushroom Thyme Frittata boasts an array of health advantages. Mushrooms are a treasure trove of essential nutrients, including vitamins like B and D, minerals like selenium, and powerful antioxidants. They can bolster your immune system, support heart health, and aid in weight management. Thyme, on the other hand, is renowned for its anti-inflammatory properties and is packed with vitamins and antioxidants, contributing to improved digestion and overall well-being.

PREPARATION

Creating this culinary masterpiece is a breeze. Start by sautéing sliced mushrooms in a skillet until they're tender and golden brown. Then, whisk together eggs, fresh thyme leaves, and a touch of grated cheese. Pour this mixture over the mushrooms and let it cook until the edges set. Finish by transferring the skillet to the oven to let the frittata puff up and develop a delicate golden crust. In just a matter of minutes, you'll have a Mushroom Thyme Frittata ready to serve—a dish that combines gourmet flavors with a host of nutritional BENEFITS, making it an excellent addition to your culinary repertoire.

ALMOND CREAM CHEESE PANCAKES

In the realm of breakfast delights, Almond Cream Cheese Pancakes stand out as a delectable fusion of taste and healthfulness. These pancakes, beloved by many for their fluffy texture and rich flavor, offer a delightful twist to traditional breakfast fare.

BENEFITS

What sets Almond Cream Cheese Pancakes apart is their health-conscious profile. They are a smart choice for those seeking a balance between indulgence and nutrition. Almonds, a key ingredient, provide a dose of healthy fats, fiber, and protein, making these pancakes a satiating morning option. The inclusion of cream cheese not only enhances the pancakes' creaminess but also contributes to a luscious taste. Additionally, these pancakes are naturally low in carbohydrates and sugar, making them an ideal choice for individuals looking to manage their blood sugar levels.

PREPARATION

Creating Almond Cream Cheese Pancakes is a straightforward process. Begin by mixing almond flour, cream cheese, eggs, and a touch of baking powder in a bowl until you achieve a smooth, thick batter. Then, ladle the batter onto a hot, greased skillet or griddle and cook until the pancakes are golden brown on both sides. The result is a stack of pancakes that are not only visually appealing but also brimming with flavor. Serve them warm with your choice of toppings, whether it's fresh berries, a drizzle of sugar-free syrup, or a dollop of Greek yogurt.

Almond Cream Cheese Pancakes are a scrumptious and wholesome breakfast option that proves you don't have to sacrifice taste for health. With their satisfying texture and balanced nutrition, they offer a delightful way to kickstart your day while keeping your

SCRAMBLED EGGS

Scrambled eggs, a breakfast classic, offer both delectable flavors and a host of nutritional BENEFITS. This versatile dish is quick and easy to prepare, making it a perfect choice for busy mornings. The process involves whisking eggs, seasoning with a pinch of salt and pepper, and cooking them in a non-stick pan with a touch of butter or oil. The result? Soft, creamy curds that tantalize the taste buds.

Beyond their deliciousness, scrambled eggs are a nutritional powerhouse, boasting high-quality protein, essential vitamins, and minerals like vitamin B12, choline, and selenium. They promote satiety, aiding in weight management, and provide sustained energy throughout the day. Plus, the simplicity of PREPARATION allows for customization with various ingredients such as vegetables, herbs, or cheese, adding extra flavor and nutrients. Scrambled eggs exemplify a wholesome breakfast that caters to taste and health in one delightful package.

SNACKS AND SIDE

In the intricate journey of pregnancy, where every bite holds profound significance, managing gestational diabetes demands a delicate balance between nourishing both mother and baby. As expectant mothers navigate the challenges of this condition, the importance of maintaining stable blood sugar levels becomes paramount. This is where the world of "Snacks and Sides for Gestational Diabetes Diet" opens its doors—a realm where delectable and health-conscious culinary choices come together to support maternal well-being. In this guide, we embark on a flavorful exploration of snacks and side dishes specifically tailored to the needs of expectant mothers with gestational diabetes. These recipes are thoughtfully designed to harmonize with the dietary requirements of gestational diabetes while ensuring that taste and enjoyment remain at the forefront. Each bite represents a balance between nurturing the growing life within and safeguarding maternal health, promising a culinary journey that is both wholesome and satisfying during this extraordinary chapter of life.

WARM QUINOA TABBOULEH SALAD

Warm Quinoa Tabbouleh Salad is a vibrant and nutritious dish that combines the wholesome goodness of quinoa with the fresh flavors of traditional Middle Eastern tabbouleh. This fusion of ingredients not only tantalizes the taste buds but also offers a multitude of health BENEFITS. As a warm and satisfying salad option, it is particularly appealing for those seeking a hearty yet nutritious meal. Let's delve into the BENEFITS and PREPARATION of this delightful dish.

BENEFITS

1. Rich in Protein Quinoa is renowned for its complete protein profile, making it an excellent choice for vegetarians and vegans. It helps maintain muscle health and provides sustained energy.

2. Abundant Fiber Quinoa and fresh vegetables in tabbouleh are fiber-rich, aiding digestion, promoting a feeling of fullness, and regulating blood sugar levels.

3. Packed with Nutrients This salad is loaded with vitamins, minerals, and antioxidants from ingredients like parsley, tomatoes, and lemon juice, which support overall health.

4. Low-Glycemic The low-glycemic index of quinoa helps stabilize blood sugar levels, making it suitable for individuals with diabetes or gestational diabetes.

5. Heart-Healthy The combination of healthy fats from olive oil and fiber from vegetables contributes to heart health by reducing cholesterol levels.

PREPARATION

1. Cook Quinoa Rinse 1 cup of quinoa thoroughly. Combine with 2 cups of water in a saucepan and bring to a boil. Reduce heat, cover, and simmer for 15-20 minutes until the quinoa absorbs the water. Let it cool slightly.

2. Prepare Vegetables Dice cucumbers, tomatoes, and red onions finely. Chop fresh parsley and mint leaves.

3. Combine Ingredients In a large bowl, mix the cooked quinoa, diced vegetables, and herbs.

4. Dressing Prepare a dressing by combining extra-virgin olive oil, lemon juice, salt, and pepper

GARLIC SAUTÉED GREENS

Garlic sautéed greens are a culinary revelation that transforms humble leafy vegetables into a delectable and nutritious dish. This simple yet flavorful PREPARATION offers a vibrant fusion of garlic's pungent aroma and the earthy freshness of greens. Beyond its tantalizing taste, this dish boasts a host of health BENEFITS and versatility in the kitchen, making it a staple in many cuisines around the world.

BENEFITS

The BENEFITS of garlic sautéed greens extend far beyond their delicious flavor. First and foremost, they are a nutritional powerhouse. Leafy greens such as spinach, kale, or collard greens are rich in vitamins A, C, and K, as well as essential minerals like iron and calcium. Garlic, renowned for its medicinal properties, adds anti-inflammatory and immune-boosting qualities to the mix. Moreover, this dish is a low-calorie option that supports weight management and helps regulate blood sugar levels. The fiber content aids digestion, while the antioxidants in greens contribute to overall well-being. Consuming garlic sautéed greens can also promote heart health by reducing cholesterol levels. Additionally, this dish is a versatile side that pairs harmoniously with various main courses, adding a burst of flavor and nutrients to your meals.

PREPARATION

To prepare garlic sautéed greens, start by washing and chopping your choice of leafy greens (spinach, kale, chard, or collard greens work well). In a pan, heat a small amount of olive oil over medium heat, then add minced garlic, allowing it to infuse the oil with its aroma. Next, toss in the greens, season with a pinch of salt and pepper, and sauté until they wilt and become tender. For added zest, consider incorporating a squeeze of lemon juice or a sprinkle of red pepper flakes. The entire process takes only minutes, yielding a flavorful, nutrient-rich side dish that pairs wonderfully with various proteins or grains. Garlic sautéed greens are a delightful way to elevate your daily dose of vitamins and minerals while tantalizing your taste buds.

SEEDING COCONUT SNACK BARS

Seeding Coconut Snack Bars are a delightful fusion of flavor and nutrition, offering a delicious and wholesome snack option for health-conscious individuals. These bars are not only a treat for your taste buds but also a convenient way to incorporate essential nutrients into your diet. Packed with seeds, coconut, and other wholesome ingredients, these snack bars are a smart choice for those seeking a satisfying and energizing snack.

BENEFITS

Seeding Coconut Snack Bars are a nutritional powerhouse. They are rich in fiber, providing a steady release of energy to keep you fueled throughout the day. The seeds, such as chia, flax, and pumpkin seeds, deliver a dose of heart-healthy fats and essential minerals like magnesium and zinc. Additionally, coconut adds a touch of natural sweetness and healthy fats while enhancing the bars' texture and flavor. These snack bars are not only satisfying but also contribute to better digestion, improved heart health, and enhanced overall well-being.

PREPARATION

Creating Seeding Coconut Snack Bars at home is a straightforward and rewarding process. Begin by combining a mixture of seeds (chia, flax, pumpkin, etc.) with shredded coconut, oats, and a touch of honey or maple syrup for sweetness. Add a binding agent like nut butter and mix until the ingredients form a cohesive mixture. Press this mixture into a baking pan, refrigerate until firm, and then cut it into convenient bars. The result is a batch of homemade snack bars that are not only delicious but also tailored to your taste and dietary preferences. Whether you're looking for a quick energy boost or a satisfying on-the-go snack, these Seeding Coconut Snack Bars are a tasty and nutritious choice that you can enjoy guilt-free.

LEMON PARMESAN ROASTED BROCCOLI

When it comes to transforming a humble vegetable into a culinary masterpiece, Lemon Parmesan Roasted Broccoli stands as a shining example. This vibrant dish not only tantalizes the taste buds but also boasts a plethora of health BENEFITS that make it a star in any meal lineup.

BENEFITS

Roasted to perfection, broccoli retains its vibrant green hue and crisp texture, while the addition of zesty lemon and savory Parmesan elevates it to new heights. Beyond its delectable taste, this dish is a nutritional powerhouse. Broccoli is brimming with vitamins, minerals, and fiber, promoting digestive health and bolstering the immune system. The citrusy infusion of lemon provides a dose of vitamin C, while Parmesan adds a satisfying umami kick and a dose of protein and calcium.

PREPARATION

Creating this culinary delight is a straightforward process. Begin by preheating your oven and preparing a baking sheet with parchment paper. Cut fresh broccoli into florets and arrange them on the baking sheet. Drizzle with olive oil, ensuring each floret is lightly coated, and season with salt and pepper to taste. Squeeze fresh lemon juice over the broccoli, adding a refreshing citrus zing. Roast in the oven until the broccoli edges turn golden and crispy. Before serving, sprinkle with grated Parmesan for a burst of savory flavor.

TUSCAN ZUCCHINI SKILLET

Tuscan Zucchini Skillet is A Taste of Mediterranean Wellness. It is more than just a delicious dish; it's a gateway to savoring the wholesome flavors of the Mediterranean while reaping a host of health BENEFITS. This vibrant and nutritious creation combines the bounty of fresh zucchini with the aromatic essence of Tuscan herbs and spices, offering a mouthwatering experience that delights the taste buds and nourishes the body.

BENEFITS

Beyond its delightful taste, this skillet dish is brimming with health advantages. Zucchini, the star ingredient, is a low-calorie, high-fiber vegetable that supports digestive health and provides essential vitamins and minerals. The Mediterranean-inspired seasonings, like oregano and garlic, not only enhance the flavor but also offer antioxidant properties that promote overall well-being. This dish's light and balanced profile make it an ideal choice for those seeking weight management and improved heart health, as it's low in saturated fats and rich in dietary fiber.

PREPARATION

Creating this Tuscan Zucchini Skillet is a breeze. Begin by slicing fresh zucchini into rounds and sautéing them in olive oil until they become tender and slightly golden. Next, infuse the dish with the aromatic combination of garlic, dried oregano, and red pepper flakes, adding a touch of crushed tomatoes for depth of flavor. Allow these ingredients to meld together, transforming the zucchini into a Mediterranean masterpiece. Finish with a sprinkle of fresh basil leaves and a drizzle of extra-virgin olive oil for an authentic Tuscan touch. You can savor the essence of the Mediterranean diet with the Tuscan Zucchini Skillet a dish that not only pleases the palate but also promotes your well-being, making it a delightful addition to your culinary repertoire.

SOUP AND SALADS

Amidst this culinary journey, few dishes prove as versatile, healthful, and downright delicious as soups and salads. Welcome to a world where flavors flourish and nutrients shine, where every spoonful or forkful is a step towards better health for both you and your growing baby. In this comprehensive guide to soups and salads tailored for a gestational diabetes diet, we will talk on a flavorful exploration, embracing the art of crafting delectable and blood sugar-friendly creations. From hearty soups brimming with wholesome ingredients to vibrant salads bursting with color and vitality, these recipes not only cater to your nutritional needs but also celebrate the joy of eating well. We delve into the intricacies of ingredient selection, mindful portioning, and culinary creativity, ensuring that every meal is a delightful and nourishing experience on your gestational diabetes journey.

GREEN AND EGG SALAD

Green and Egg Salad is a delectable and nutrient-packed dish that offers a myriad of BENEFITS for your health and taste buds alike. Combining the freshness of vibrant greens with the protein punch of eggs, this salad is a symphony of flavors and textures that is not only satisfying but also incredibly nourishing.

BENEFITS

This salad boasts an array of health BENEFITS. The leafy greens, such as spinach and kale, are rich in vitamins, minerals, and fiber, promoting digestive health and providing essential nutrients for pregnancy. Eggs, on the other hand, are a protein powerhouse, aiding in fetal development and keeping you feeling full and energized. The combination of greens and eggs also offers a substantial dose of antioxidants and folate, crucial for combating inflammation and supporting neural tube development in your growing baby.

PREPARATION

Creating this nutritious dish is a breeze. Begin by washing and drying your choice of greens, whether it's spinach, kale, arugula, or a mix. Hard boil eggs, then slice or chop them into bite-sized pieces. Toss the greens and eggs together in a bowl. You can add other ingredients like cherry tomatoes, cucumbers, or avocado for extra flavor and nutrients. Top it off with a light vinaigrette dressing or a creamy yogurt-based sauce for a delightful finishing touch. This Green and Egg Salad is not only a tasty addition to your gestational diabetes diet but also a quick and easy meal to prepare, ensuring that you can savor both convenience and health in every bite.

CHICKEN CAULIFLOWER RICE BOWLS

Chicken Cauliflower Rice Bowls are a flavorful and nutritious meal that perfectly embodies the principles of a balanced and health-conscious diet. This dish not only delivers on taste but also offers a range of BENEFITS for those seeking a wholesome and satisfying option. From its low-carb profile to its high protein content, it's an ideal choice for individuals aiming to manage their weight, control blood sugar levels, or simply enjoy a delicious, guilt-free meal.

BENEFITS

One of the standout BENEFITS of Chicken Cauliflower Rice Bowls is its low carbohydrate content, which makes it a valuable addition to diets aimed at managing conditions like diabetes or supporting weight loss goals. Cauliflower rice, a versatile substitute for traditional rice, is low in calories and carbs, helping stabilize blood sugar levels. Chicken, a lean source of protein, promotes satiety and muscle maintenance. Moreover, this dish is packed with essential vitamins, minerals, and fiber, courtesy of colorful vegetables. Its customizable nature allows for various seasonings and toppings to suit individual tastes and dietary needs.

PREPARATION

Preparing Chicken Cauliflower Rice Bowls is both straightforward and rewarding. Begin by marinating chicken breast in your preferred seasonings, then cook until it's tender and succulent. Meanwhile, pulse cauliflower florets in a food processor to create the rice-like texture. Sauté the cauliflower rice with aromatic vegetables like bell peppers, onions, and garlic. Assemble your bowls with a generous serving of cauliflower rice, slices of the cooked chicken, and a medley of fresh veggies. Finish with a drizzle of your favorite low-sugar sauce or dressing for an added burst of flavor. The result is a wholesome and visually appealing meal that's as enjoyable to make as it is to savor.

COCONUT CHICKEN SOUP

Coconut chicken soup, known for its delightful fusion of flavors and nourishing qualities, is a beloved dish that transcends culinary boundaries. This aromatic and savory soup brings together the creamy richness of coconut milk, the zest of Thai or Asian spices, and the heartiness of tender chicken to create a harmonious and comforting bowl of goodness. Beyond its delectable taste, coconut chicken soup offers a range of health BENEFITS. The coconut milk lends a creamy texture while being a source of healthy fats. It's also a fantastic source of medium-chain triglycerides (MCTs), known for their quick energy release. The chicken provides a generous dose of lean protein, essential for tissue repair and immune support.

PREPARATION of this soup is a delightful journey in itself. Start by simmering chicken in a flavorful broth infused with lemongrass, ginger, and garlic. Then, add the creamy coconut milk, allowing the flavors to meld together. A burst of lime juice adds a zesty twist, and a garnish of fresh herbs, such as cilantro and basil, imparts a fragrant finish. Whether enjoyed as a light and satisfying meal or a comforting bowl on a chilly day, coconut chicken soup combines the exotic allure of coconut with the wholesomeness of chicken, making it a flavorful and nutritious addition to any menu.

CREAMY CAULIFLOWER SOUP

Creamy cauliflower soup, a velvety and wholesome delight, stands as a testament to the delightful possibilities of nutritious eating. This delectable dish not only tickles the taste buds but also offers a plethora of BENEFITS for those seeking a health-conscious option.

BENEFITS

Creamy cauliflower soup is a nutritional powerhouse, especially for individuals with dietary restrictions like those managing gestational diabetes. This soup is naturally low in carbohydrates and sugars, making it a smart choice to help regulate blood sugar levels. It's also an excellent source of vitamins and minerals, including vitamin C, vitamin K, and folate, essential for the health of both mother and baby during pregnancy. Moreover, cauliflower contains fiber, promoting digestive health and aiding in satiety.

PREPARATION

Creating this soup is a straightforward and rewarding process. Start by sautéing onions and garlic in a little olive oil until they turn translucent. Add cauliflower florets and vegetable broth, then let them simmer until the cauliflower is tender. After blending the mixture until smooth, stir in a touch of low-fat milk or yogurt for creaminess. Season with herbs and spices of your choice, such as thyme or nutmeg, and a pinch of salt and pepper. Finish with a garnish of fresh herbs or a sprinkle of grated Parmesan for extra flavor. The result is a lusciously smooth and guilt-free soup, perfect for soothing your palate while supporting your gestational diabetes dietary goals.

BARBECUE CHICKEN WRAPS

Barbecue chicken wraps, a beloved culinary creation, offer a harmonious fusion of smoky, savory flavors and wholesome ingredients. These delicious wraps are not only a treat for the taste buds but also provide numerous BENEFITS for those seeking a balanced and satisfying meal.

BENEFITS

Barbecue chicken wraps are a superb choice for those looking to enjoy a satisfying and nutritious meal. Grilled chicken, a key ingredient, supplies lean protein, promoting muscle health and satiety. The barbecue sauce, when chosen wisely, adds a burst of flavor without excessive sugar or unhealthy additives. Vegetables like crisp lettuce, juicy tomatoes, and crunchy bell peppers contribute essential vitamins, fiber, and antioxidants. Wrapping it all in a whole-grain tortilla ensures a good dose of complex carbohydrates, aiding in sustained energy levels.

PREPARATION

Creating these delectable wraps is a straightforward and rewarding process. Begin by marinating chicken breast pieces in a well-balanced barbecue sauce and grilling until perfectly charred and cooked through. Then, assemble your wrap by placing a generous portion of the grilled chicken on a whole-grain tortilla. Add a colorful array of fresh vegetables, such as lettuce, tomatoes, and bell peppers, for added nutrition and texture. Finally, fold the tortilla, tucking in the sides, and secure it with toothpicks if needed. Your barbecue chicken wrap is now ready to enjoy, either as a quick lunch or a delightful dinner option.

BAKED FALAFEL

Baked falafel, a beloved Middle Eastern delight, offers a delectable fusion of flavors and health BENEFITS. These bite-sized, crispy morsels of chickpea goodness are a vegetarian's delight, providing a satisfying alternative to their deep-fried counterparts. Beyond their delicious taste and versatility, baked falafel comes with a host of advantages for those seeking a wholesome and nutritious meal.

BENEFITS

Baked falafel is a nutritional powerhouse. It's rich in plant-based protein, making it an excellent choice for vegetarians and vegans looking to meet their protein needs. Chickpeas, the primary ingredient, are packed with fiber, aiding digestion and promoting a feeling of fullness, which can be especially beneficial for weight management and blood sugar control. Additionally, baked falafel is lower in fat and calories compared to traditional fried falafel, making it heart-healthy and suitable for individuals watching their calorie intake.

PREPARATION

Crafting baked falafel at home is a straightforward and rewarding process. Start by soaking dried chickpeas overnight to soften them. Then, blend the chickpeas with a blend of herbs and spices, including garlic, cumin, coriander, parsley, and a touch of baking powder for fluffiness. Form the mixture into small patties and arrange them on a baking sheet. A light drizzle of olive oil ensures a crispy exterior. Bake in a preheated oven until golden brown and delightfully crunchy.

Baked falafel can be enjoyed in various ways — tucked into pita bread with fresh veggies and tahini sauce, served atop salads, or as a wholesome appetizer. Its health BENEFITS, ease of

PREPARATION, and scrumptious taste make it a delightful addition to any diet, satisfying both your palate and your nutritional needs.

SOUTHWESTERN CHOPPED SALAD

The Southwestern Chopped Salad is a culinary masterpiece that marries the vibrant flavors of the American Southwest with the wholesome goodness of fresh vegetables. This salad not only tantalizes the taste buds but also provides a plethora of health BENEFITS, making it a perfect choice for those seeking a nourishing and delicious meal. Its PREPARATION is a breeze, making it an ideal addition to your menu for a quick, satisfying, and nutrient-packed dining experience.

BENEFITS

The Southwestern Chopped Salad is a nutritional powerhouse. It boasts a generous serving of crisp lettuce, tomatoes, bell peppers, and corn, providing an abundance of vitamins, minerals, and dietary fiber that support overall health. Black beans and grilled chicken or tofu add a protein punch, aiding in muscle development and keeping you feeling full and satisfied. The addition of avocado contributes heart-healthy monounsaturated fats while the zesty dressing delivers a burst of flavor with minimal added sugar and sodium. This salad is an excellent choice for managing weight and blood sugar levels, making it particularly suitable for those with diabetes or anyone looking to adopt a healthier eating pattern.

PREPARATION

Creating this Southwestern Chopped Salad is a straightforward and enjoyable process. Begin by chopping a mix of fresh vegetables, such as romaine lettuce, tomatoes, bell peppers, and red onions, into bite-sized pieces. Add a cup of black beans, a handful of grilled chicken or tofu for protein, and a sliced avocado for creaminess and healthy fats. Finish with a sprinkling of corn kernels and a drizzle of a zesty, low-sugar dressing, like a lime vinaigrette or a salsa-infused option. Toss it all together, and your Southwestern Chopped Salad is ready to be savored. It's a delightful, filling, and health-conscious meal that embraces the flavors of the Southwest while contributing to your well-being.

MEATLESS – MEALS

The Meatless Meals for Gestational Diabetes Diet is a comprehensive guide designed to support expectant mothers in navigating this delicate balance. During this transformative time, the health and well-being of both mother and baby take center stage, making dietary choices of paramount importance. This book is a valuable resource, offering a diverse array of meatless meal options tailored specifically to the unique dietary requirements of women dealing with gestational diabetes. Within these pages, you'll find a rich tapestry of flavorful and nutrient-packed recipes, carefully curated to help stabilize blood sugar levels while savoring a wide range of delicious, meatless dishes. Whether you're a vegetarian, vegan, or simply looking to reduce meat consumption during pregnancy, this is your trusted companion on the path to a healthy and thriving pregnancy journey.

VEGAN BURRITO BOWL

The Vegan Burrito Bowl is a culinary masterpiece that combines the vibrant flavors of Mexican cuisine with the health-conscious choices of a vegan diet. This delicious dish offers a plethora of BENEFITS for both your taste buds and your well-being. Bursting with color and packed with

essential nutrients, the Vegan Burrito Bowl is a
celebration of plant-based goodness.

BENEFITS

One of the primary advantages of indulging in a
Vegan Burrito Bowl is its healthful nature. This
meal is rich in fiber, thanks to the abundance of
beans, whole grains, and fresh vegetables, aiding
digestion and promoting a feeling of fullness.
Additionally, it's a treasure trove of vitamins and
minerals, providing a boost to your immune system
and overall vitality. As a vegan option, it is
inherently low in saturated fats and cholesterol,
contributing to heart health. Moreover, the Vegan
Burrito Bowl aligns with sustainable eating
practices, reducing your carbon footprint while
nourishing your body.

PREPARATION

Creating a Vegan Burrito Bowl is a straightforward
and customizable process. Begin with a base of
cooked brown rice or quinoa. Add black beans or
pinto beans for protein and fiber. Load up on
colorful vegetables like bell peppers, tomatoes,

corn, and avocado for vitamins and flavor. Spice it up with salsa or a zesty lime dressing. Top it off with cilantro, jalapeños, and a sprinkle of vegan cheese or nutritional yeast for that extra flair. The beauty of this dish lies in its adaptability; you can tailor it to your taste and dietary preferences.

EDAMAME SUCCOTASH

Edamame succotash is a vibrant and nutritious dish that combines the delightful flavors of edamame beans, colorful vegetables, and aromatic seasonings. It not only tantalizes your taste buds but also offers a multitude of health BENEFITS, making it a smart addition to your culinary repertoire.

BENEFITS

Edamame succotash is a nutritional powerhouse. Edamame, young soybeans, are rich in plant-based protein, fiber, and essential vitamins and minerals. The combination of edamame with corn, bell peppers, and other vegetables creates a symphony of colors and nutrients. This dish is not only delicious but also provides antioxidants, which can help combat oxidative stress and inflammation.

Moreover, the fiber content promotes digestive health and helps regulate blood sugar levels, making it a suitable choice for those watching their glycemic index.

PREPARATION

Creating edamame succotash is a straightforward and enjoyable process. Start by cooking shelled edamame in boiling water for a few minutes until tender. Then, sauté them with a mix of corn kernels, bell peppers, onions, and your choice of seasoning. A dash of olive oil and some fresh herbs can elevate the flavors. The result is a visually appealing and nutritionally dense side dish that pairs wonderfully with a variety of main courses.

SUGAR AND VEGETABLE PILAF

Sugar and vegetable pilaf, a delightful fusion of natural sweetness and savory goodness, offers a unique and flavorful twist to traditional rice dishes. This delectable dish combines the natural sweetness of caramelized sugar with a medley of fresh, colorful vegetables, creating a symphony of tastes and textures that can elevate any mealtime experience.

BENEFITS

1. Balanced Flavor Profile Sugar adds a touch of sweetness that perfectly balances the savory notes of the vegetables and rice, resulting in a harmonious and satisfying flavor profile.

2. Nutrient-Rich The addition of vegetables not only enhances the taste but also boosts the nutritional value of the dish. You'll enjoy vitamins, minerals, and fiber from the vegetables, promoting overall well-being.

3. Versatility Sugar and vegetable pilaf can be customized to suit various dietary preferences. It can be prepared as a vegetarian or vegan option, and you can incorporate your favorite vegetables for added personalization.

PREPARATION

To prepare this delectable pilaf, start by caramelizing sugar in a pan until it turns a beautiful golden brown. Then, add a medley of diced vegetables like bell peppers, carrots, and peas, sautéing them until they become tender and flavorful. Finally, mix in cooked rice, allowing it to absorb the delightful combination of sweet and savory flavors.

Sugar and vegetable pilaf is not only a feast for the taste buds but also a visually appealing addition to your dining table. Whether served as a side dish or a main course, it's sure to delight your senses

TOFU BROCCOLI SKILLET

The Tofu Broccoli Skillet is a delightful culinary creation that not only tantalizes your taste buds but also delivers a powerful punch of health BENEFITS. This easy-to-make dish combines the versatility of tofu with the vibrant goodness of broccoli, resulting in a nutritious and flavorful meal that's perfect for vegetarians and vegans alike.

BENEFITS

One of the standout BENEFITS of the Tofu Broccoli
Skillet is its nutritional prowess. Tofu, a soy-based
protein, offers a plant-powered protein source
that's rich in essential amino acids, making it a
fantastic choice for muscle maintenance and
overall well-being. Broccoli, on the other hand, is a
nutritional powerhouse, packed with vitamins,
fiber, and antioxidants that support immune health
and digestion. Together, they form a dynamic duo
that can aid in weight management, enhance bone
health, and lower the risk of chronic diseases.

PREPARATION

Creating this savory skillet dish is a breeze. Begin by
marinating cubed tofu in a flavorful sauce, allowing
it to absorb the delicious flavors. Then, sauté it
with broccoli florets and your choice of aromatic
ingredients such as garlic, ginger, or sesame oil for
an extra layer of taste. The result is a vibrant,
protein-packed meal that can be enjoyed as a main
course or paired with rice, noodles, or quinoa for a
complete and satisfying dining experience.
Whether you're seeking a quick weeknight dinner
or a nutritious addition to your meatless
repertoire, the Tofu Broccoli Skillet is a culinary

masterpiece that embodies the essence of wholesome, delicious eating.

SEAFOOD AND POULTRY

Navigating the delicate balance of a gestational diabetes diet can be both a challenge and an opportunity for expectant mothers. We set sail into the realm of seafood and poultry, two versatile and nutritious categories that can play a pivotal role in maintaining stable blood sugar levels during pregnancy. As gestational diabetes demands thoughtful dietary choices, these protein-rich options become invaluable allies, providing essential nutrients while helping manage glucose levels. In this guide, we embark on a flavorful exploration, offering an array of tantalizing recipes that not only adhere to the dietary restrictions of gestational diabetes but also celebrate the joy of eating. From succulent salmon to tender chicken, we present dishes that balance taste and nutrition, ensuring that every meal is a delightful and health-conscious experience for both mother and baby. Whether you're seeking inspiration for weekday dinners or special occasions, our seafood and poultry recipes are here to empower you in your journey to a healthy and fulfilling pregnancy.

CRAB CAKES

Crab cakes, a beloved coastal delicacy, are more than just a culinary delight; they represent a delectable fusion of flavors and a wholesome seafood choice. These savory patties, typically made from crab meat, breadcrumbs, and an array of herbs and seasonings, offer numerous BENEFITS to both the palate and the body.

BENEFITS

Crab cakes are a treasure trove of BENEFITS. Firstly, they are a rich source of lean protein, essential for muscle development and overall health. The crab meat provides omega-3 fatty acids, promoting heart health and reducing inflammation. Additionally, they are relatively low in saturated fats, making them an excellent choice for those watching their cholesterol levels. Crab cakes are also abundant in essential vitamins and minerals, including vitamin B12, zinc, and selenium, which support immunity and cellular function.

PREPARATIONs

Crafting the perfect crab cake involves a delicate balance of flavors and textures. Begin with fresh, high-quality crab meat, whether it's lump crab, claw meat, or a combination. Mix it with breadcrumbs (preferably whole-grain for added fiber), eggs to bind, and a medley of seasonings such as Old Bay, Worcestershire sauce, and fresh herbs like parsley. Form the mixture into patties and lightly pan-fry them in a small amount of heart-healthy oil until golden brown and crispy.

Crab cakes are versatile; they can be served as an appetizer, a main course, or even tucked into sandwiches. Pair them with a zesty remoulade sauce, a squeeze of lemon, or a refreshing salad for a delightful meal that celebrates the flavors of the sea. With their nutritional BENEFITS and culinary versatility, crab cakes are a seafood sensation worth savoring.

ROASTED RATATOUILLE GOLD

Roasted Ratatouille Gold, a golden twist on the classic Provençal dish, embodies a harmonious fusion of flavors, vibrant colors, and exceptional health BENEFITS. This delectable creation is not only a culinary masterpiece but also a nutritional powerhouse that deserves a special place in your kitchen.

The BENEFITS Roasted Ratatouille Gold offers a plethora of BENEFITS for both your taste buds and your well-being. Bursting with a medley of vegetables, including tomatoes, bell peppers, eggplants, and zucchini, it's rich in antioxidants, vitamins, and dietary fiber. These components contribute to a strengthened immune system, improved digestion, and reduced risk of chronic diseases. Furthermore, this dish is remarkably low in calories and saturated fats, making it an excellent choice for those aiming to maintain a healthy weight.

PREPARATION Creating Roasted Ratatouille Gold is a culinary adventure that rewards your efforts with a symphony of flavors. Start by slicing the vegetables into thin, uniform rounds. Then, arrange them in an overlapping pattern in a baking dish, drizzle with olive oil, and season with aromatic herbs like thyme and rosemary. Roast until the vegetables turn tender and develop a captivating golden hue. The result is a visually stunning and mouthwatering dish that can be enjoyed as a side, a topping for pasta, or even a standalone entrée.

JUICY TURKEY BURGERS

Juicy turkey burgers offer a delicious departure from traditional beef patties, bringing a bounty of BENEFITS to your plate. These succulent creations not only tantalize your taste buds but also align seamlessly with a health-conscious lifestyle. Prepared with lean ground turkey, they are naturally lower in saturated fat, making them heart-friendly and ideal for those seeking a leaner protein source.

The PREPARATION of juicy turkey burgers is a breeze. Begin with lean ground turkey meat, typically a blend of white and dark meat, which ensures moisture and flavor. Enhance the patty's juiciness by incorporating ingredients like finely chopped onions, garlic, and breadcrumbs. Seasonings such as fresh herbs, spices, and a dash of Worcestershire sauce add depth and zest.

To maximize tenderness and juiciness, avoid overmixing the ingredients and handle the meat gently. Shape the patties to your preferred thickness, then grill, pan-fry, or bake them to perfection. The result? Burgers that are not only bursting with flavor but also juicier and more nutritious than their beef counterparts. Serve them on whole-grain buns with your favorite toppings, and you'll savor a guilt-free indulgence that keeps you nourished and satisfied.

TILAPIA TACOS WITH AVO-CADO

Tilapia tacos with avo-cado offer a mouthwatering and nutritious culinary journey that combines the goodness of tilapia fish with the creamy richness of avocado. These tacos not only tantalize your taste buds but also provide a host of health BENEFITS, making them a perfect addition to your menu.

BENEFITS

Tilapia, a mild and lean white fish, is a great source of protein and low in saturated fats, making it an excellent choice for heart health. Meanwhile, avocados contribute healthy fats, fiber, and an abundance of vitamins and minerals, including potassium. This combination not only satisfies your hunger but also promotes overall well-being.

PREPARATION

Creating tilapia tacos with avo-cado is a straightforward process. Begin by seasoning and grilling tilapia fillets until they are tender and flaky. While the fish cooks, prepare a creamy avocado salsa by mashing ripe avocados and blending them with lime juice, diced tomatoes, onions, and cilantro. Assemble your tacos by placing a generous portion of grilled tilapia in warm corn tortillas, topping them with the avocado salsa, and garnishing with extra lime wedges and fresh herbs.

These tilapia tacos with avo-cado are a delightful combination of textures and flavors, offering a burst of freshness and nutrition in every bite. Enjoy the satisfaction of a delicious meal while knowing that you're fueling your body with ingredients that support your health and well-being.

MEAT MEALS

In the delicate journey of pregnancy, managing gestational diabetes can be a daunting task, but it's also an opportunity to embrace a wholesome and nourishing diet that supports both the mother and the growing baby. Welcome to the world of "Meat Meals for Gestational Diabetes Diet," a culinary adventure designed to provide expecting mothers with a delectable array of meat-based dishes tailored to meet the specific dietary needs of gestational diabetes. In this carefully curated collection, we will explore how the rich and satisfying flavors of meats can be harnessed to create balanced and blood sugar-friendly meals. From succulent poultry to tender cuts of beef and lamb, we will uncover recipes that not only satisfy your taste buds but also help regulate blood glucose levels during pregnancy. Join us on this culinary journey as we celebrate the joy of eating well and nurturing your health during this special time.

PORK CUTLETS

Pork cutlets, a culinary gem cherished by food enthusiasts worldwide, offer a delectable experience with a perfect blend of flavor and tenderness. These thin slices of pork loin or tenderloin are not only a treat for your taste buds but also bring numerous BENEFITS to your dining table.

BENEFITS

1. Lean Protein Pork cutlets are a lean source of protein, essential for muscle development and overall health. They offer a satisfying, meaty texture without excessive fat content.

2. Rich in Vitamins and Minerals These cuts provide a wealth of essential nutrients like vitamin B6, niacin, phosphorus, and selenium, promoting optimal body function and vitality.

3. Versatility Pork cutlets are remarkably versatile, adapting to various culinary styles and flavors. They can be breaded and pan-fried, grilled, or baked, making them suitable for a wide range of dishes.

PREPARATIONs

Preparing succulent pork cutlets is an art that begins with selecting quality meat. Trim excess fat and pound the slices to an even thickness for consistent cooking. Season with your favorite herbs and spices, and then choose from a variety of cooking methods. For a crispy texture, dredge them in breadcrumbs and pan-fry until golden brown. Alternatively, marinate and grill for a smoky, flavorful profile. Pair with your preferred side dishes, from mashed potatoes to vibrant salads, for a memorable meal that elevates the humble pork cutlet into a culinary masterpiece. Whether you savor them as a quick weeknight dinner or as the centerpiece of a special occasion, pork cutlets promise a delightful dining experience that satisfies both your palate and your nutrition needs.

MUSTARD PORK

Mustard pork is a delectable culinary creation that combines the rich flavors of pork with the bold and tangy essence of mustard. Beyond its irresistible taste, this dish offers a multitude of BENEFITS, making it a favorite on many dinner tables.

BENEFITS

1. Protein-Rich Pork is a fantastic source of high-quality protein, essential for muscle growth and repair. It provides the body with the necessary amino acids during digestion.

2. Nutrient Density Pork is rich in vitamins and minerals, including B vitamins like B12 and niacin, which play crucial roles in energy metabolism and overall health.

3. Mustard's Zing Mustard adds a flavorful kick to the dish without the need for excessive salt or unhealthy fats, making it a heart-healthy option.

PREPARATION

Creating mustard pork is a straightforward process. Start by marinating pork chops or tenderloin in a mixture of Dijon or whole-grain mustard, olive oil, garlic, and herbs. Allow the flavors to meld for at least 30 minutes or longer for a more intense taste. Then, sear the pork in a hot skillet until it's beautifully caramelized and cooked to perfection. Serve with a side of vegetables or a simple salad for a balanced meal that tantalizes the taste buds while nourishing the body. Mustard pork is not only a culinary delight but also a nutritious addition to your dining repertoire.

PORK SPAGHETTI WITH MUSHROOM SAUCE

Indulge in a culinary journey that marries the savory goodness of pork with the earthy richness of mushroom sauce in this delightful Pork Spaghetti with Mushroom Sauce recipe. Beyond its tantalizing taste, this dish offers a medley of BENEFITS that make it a must-try for any food enthusiast.

BENEFITS

1. Protein-Packed Pleasure Pork brings a generous dose of high-quality protein to the table, essential for muscle development and overall body function. During pregnancy or simply as part of a balanced diet, protein is crucial.

2. Iron Enrichment Pork is a valuable source of heme iron, which is readily absorbed by the body. This is particularly important for pregnant women,

as iron aids in carrying oxygen to both the mother and the growing fetus.

3. Folate-Rich Mushrooms Mushrooms in the sauce contribute folate, a vital B-vitamin that supports fetal neural development.

PREPARATION

1. Ingredients Gather pork loin slices, spaghetti, mushrooms, onions, garlic, chicken broth, cream, Parmesan cheese, olive oil, salt, pepper, and fresh herbs.

2. Cooking Pork Season pork slices with salt and pepper, then sauté them in olive oil until golden brown. Set aside.

3. Mushroom Sauce In the same pan, add sliced mushrooms, onions, and garlic. Cook until they soften. Pour in chicken broth, cream, and

Parmesan cheese, simmering until the sauce thickens. Season to taste.

4. Combining Toss cooked spaghetti with the mushroom sauce and top with the succulent pork slices.

5. Garnish Finish with fresh herbs like parsley or basil for a burst of color and flavor.

This Pork Spaghetti with Mushroom Sauce isn't just a feast for the senses; it's a nutrient-packed dish, perfect for prenatal nutrition. Whether you're an expectant mother or simply a lover of exquisite flavors, this recipe promises to satisfy both your taste buds and your dietary needs.

BEEF STEW

Beef stew, a timeless culinary classic, transcends mere sustenance; it embodies comfort and tradition in a single bowl. Beyond its delicious aroma and rich flavors, beef stew boasts a range of healthful BENEFITS that make it a staple in many households. This beloved dish combines tender cuts of beef with an assortment of vegetables, simmered to perfection in a savory broth. Its versatility and nutritional value make it a cherished favorite for both nourishing family dinners and special occasions.

BENEFITS

1. Nutrient-Rich Beef stew is a treasure trove of essential nutrients, offering high-quality protein, vitamins like B-complex and C, and minerals such as iron and zinc. These nutrients contribute to muscle health, immune support, and overall vitality.

2. Fiber and Vegetables The addition of vegetables like carrots, potatoes, and celery introduces dietary fiber, promoting digestive health and providing essential vitamins and antioxidants. These components contribute to improved digestion and overall well-being.

3. Sustained Energy The combination of protein, complex carbohydrates from vegetables, and

healthy fats from the broth creates a balanced meal that sustains energy levels and helps manage blood sugar.

PREPARATIONs

Creating a delectable beef stew requires patience, but the process is simple. Start by browning beef cubes in a hot pot to enhance flavor. Add onions, garlic, and a medley of vegetables. Pour in a combination of broth and diced tomatoes, then season with herbs and spices like thyme, rosemary, and bay leaves. Simmer gently over low heat for hours, allowing the flavors to meld, and the meat to become tender. The result is a hearty, nutritious, and soul-soothing meal that can be enjoyed as a stand-alone dish or paired with crusty bread for a complete dining experience.

SPICY NACHO SKILLET

Introducing the Spicy Nacho Skillet, a culinary delight that effortlessly combines bold flavors, convenience, and nutritional BENEFITS into one hearty dish. This spicy twist on the classic nacho recipe is not only a treat for your taste buds but also offers several advantages for those seeking a satisfying and spicy meal.

BENEFITS

1. Rich in Protein The Spicy Nacho Skillet packs a protein punch, thanks to ingredients like lean ground meat or plant-based alternatives. Protein is essential for muscle health and helps keep you feeling full and satisfied.

2. Flavor Explosion This dish is a flavor explosion, with the heat of spices, the creaminess of cheese, and the crunch of nacho chips coming together in perfect harmony.

3. Customizable Tailor it to your preferences by choosing your level of spiciness, protein source, and toppings. Load it up with vegetables for added nutrition.

PREPARATION

Creating a Spicy Nacho Skillet is a breeze. Start by browning your choice of ground meat or meat substitute in a skillet. Then, add spicy seasonings like chili powder, cumin, and paprika for that irresistible kick. Layer on some nacho chips and sprinkle generously with shredded cheese. Pop the skillet in the oven until the cheese is bubbly and golden. Finish with toppings like diced tomatoes, jalapeños, and fresh cilantro. Serve it hot, and watch it disappear in no time.

CHILI

Chili, a beloved dish with roots in both Texan and Mexican cuisines, stands as a testament to the power of hearty, spiced goodness. Beyond its tantalizing taste and versatility, chili offers a wealth of BENEFITS that make it a favorite among food enthusiasts.

Health BENEFITS

First and foremost, chili can be a nutritional powerhouse. Packed with protein from beans and meat (or meat alternatives), it provides sustained energy and helps maintain muscle health. Additionally, chili's signature spice, often derived from chili peppers, contains capsaicin, known for its potential metabolism-boosting properties and pain relief. Capsaicin may also aid in appetite control and weight management.

PREPARATION

Chili's PREPARATION can be as diverse as the people who make it. It starts with a flavorful base of sautéed onions and garlic, followed by the star ingredients beans, tomatoes, and your choice of meat or vegetables. Seasonings like chili powder, cumin, and paprika bring depth and heat to the dish. Simmered low and slow, chili develops its rich, complex flavors over time, making it perfect for a slow cooker or stovetop simmering.

Chili serves as a canvas for creativity, with countless variations to cater to dietary preferences and restrictions. Whether you prefer it spicy or mild, loaded with veggies or meat, chili remains a wholesome, comforting, and deeply satisfying meal that brings warmth to both the body and soul.

NATURALLY SWEET TREATS

Embarking on the journey of motherhood is a remarkable experience, filled with anticipation and joy. However, for expectant mothers diagnosed with gestational diabetes, the path to a healthy pregnancy can be accompanied by dietary challenges. Enter "Naturally Sweet Treats for Gestational Diabetes Diet," a delectable guide designed to make this journey not only manageable but also delightful. In the pages that follow, we'll explore a world of naturally sweet and nutritious culinary creations, meticulously curated to cater to the unique needs of women managing gestational diabetes. These recipes strike a harmonious balance between the necessity for glucose control and the desire for indulgence. From guilt-free desserts to satisfying snacks and wholesome meals, each offering is crafted to satiate cravings without compromising on flavor or nutritional value. Get ready to savor a collection of recipes that not only nourish both you and your growing baby but also transform your gestational diabetes diet into a pleasurable culinary adventure.

PEANUT BUTTER TRUFFLES

Peanut Butter Truffles, the delectable fusion of velvety peanut butter and rich chocolate, offer a mouthwatering treat that transcends mere confectionery. These bite-sized delights encapsulate a harmonious blend of flavors, delivering not only an exquisite sensory experience but also a host of nutritional BENEFITS.

BENEFITS

Peanut butter, the star ingredient, brings forth its nutritional prowess, boasting a hearty dose of protein, healthy fats, and essential vitamins and minerals. Its high protein content helps in satiety, making these truffles a satisfying snack. Additionally, peanut butter provides an array of nutrients, including vitamin E, magnesium, and potassium, while being a natural source of antioxidants.

These truffles, when prepared thoughtfully, can be a healthier alternative to traditional sweets, particularly for those with dietary restrictions or health-conscious individuals. The marriage of peanut butter and dark chocolate not only satisfies sweet cravings but also provides a source of antioxidants from the cocoa.

PREPARATION

Crafting Peanut Butter Truffles is an art that balances indulgence with nutrition. To create these delights, begin by mixing creamy peanut butter with a touch of honey for sweetness and a pinch of sea salt to enhance the flavors. This luscious mixture is then rolled into bite-sized balls and chilled until firm. Once set, dip each truffle into melted dark chocolate, ensuring a decadent coating. Allow them to cool until the chocolate hardens, and you're ready to savor these delectable treats.

BAKED FILLED PEARS

Baked filled pears, a delightful dessert option, marry the natural sweetness of pears with a medley of delectable fillings, resulting in a symphony of flavors that's as pleasing to the palate as it is to the eye. This dessert isn't just about indulgence; it's a nourishing treat that offers numerous BENEFITS while satisfying your sweet cravings.

BENEFITS

1. Nutrient-Rich Pears are a rich source of dietary fiber, vitamins, and minerals, including vitamin C and potassium. When baked, their natural sugars caramelize, enhancing their sweetness.

2. Fiber for Digestion The combination of pear's inherent fiber and the fillings provides digestive BENEFITS, aiding regularity and preventing blood sugar spikes.

3. Low in Calories Baking maintains the pear's natural goodness while keeping calorie counts in check, making it a guilt-free dessert option.

PREPARATION

Creating baked filled pears is a straightforward and customizable process. Start by halving and coring ripe pears, leaving a small well in the center for the filling. Popular fillings include a mixture of chopped nuts, dried fruits, honey, and spices like cinnamon. Place the filled pear halves in a baking dish, drizzle with a touch of honey or maple syrup, and bake until tender. The result is a warm, fragrant dessert that's as visually stunning as it is delicious.

Baked filled pears not only provide a delectable treat but also showcase the natural sweetness of fruit while incorporating essential nutrients. This dessert is a testament to the idea that indulgence and health-conscious choices can harmoniously coexist in your culinary repertoire.

VANILLA CHEESECAKES MOUSSE

Indulging in a delicious dessert doesn't have to mean sacrificing your commitment to a healthier lifestyle. Enter Vanilla Cheesecake Mousse, a delightful treat that not only satisfies your sweet tooth but also offers several health BENEFITS. This creamy and velvety dessert combines the rich flavors of vanilla and cheesecake while being mindful of your well-being.

BENEFITS

1. Low Sugar Content Vanilla Cheesecake Mousse is typically prepared with reduced sugar or alternative sweeteners, making it a suitable option for those watching their sugar intake, including individuals with diabetes.

2. High Protein This dessert incorporates the goodness of dairy, providing a generous dose of protein, which can help promote a feeling of fullness and support muscle health.

3. Calcium-Rich With cream cheese or yogurt as primary ingredients, this mousse offers a significant amount of calcium, crucial for maintaining strong bones and teeth.

PREPARATION

Creating Vanilla Cheesecake Mousse is a straightforward process. Begin by blending reduced-fat cream cheese or Greek yogurt with vanilla extract and a sweetener of your choice (such as stevia or honey). Fold in whipped cream or a whipped topping for a lusciously airy texture. Refrigerate until set, and garnish with fresh berries or a sprinkle of cinnamon for an extra burst of flavor.

Managing gestational diabetes through a well-balanced diet is essential for both your health and your baby's. Here's a four-week meal plan designed to help you regulate blood sugar levels while enjoying a variety of delicious and nutritious meals. Remember to consult with your healthcare provider or a registered dietitian for personalized advice and adjustments.

MEAL PLANS

Week 1:

Day 1:

- Breakfast: Scrambled eggs with spinach and whole-grain toast

- Snack: Greek yogurt with berries

- Lunch: Grilled chicken salad with mixed greens and vinaigrette dressing

- Snack: Baby carrots with hummus

- Dinner: Baked salmon with quinoa and steamed broccoli

Day 2:

- Breakfast: Oatmeal with sliced strawberries and a sprinkle of chopped nuts

- Snack: Cottage cheese with pineapple

- Lunch: Turkey and avocado wrap with a side salad

- Snack: Almonds and a small apple

- Dinner: Stir-fried tofu with mixed vegetables and brown rice

Day 3:

- Breakfast: Whole-grain pancakes with a small portion of blueberries

- Snack: Sliced cucumber with tzatziki sauce

- Lunch: Lentil soup with a side of mixed greens

- Snack: Sugar-free gelatin

- Dinner: Baked chicken breast with quinoa and roasted asparagus

Day 4:

- Breakfast: Greek yogurt parfait with low-sugar granola and raspberries

- Snack: Sliced bell peppers with guacamole

- Lunch: Spinach and feta stuffed chicken breast with a side of quinoa

- Snack: Celery sticks with peanut butter

- Dinner: Beef stir-fry with broccoli and cauliflower rice

Day 5:

- Breakfast: Scrambled egg whites with sautéed spinach and whole-grain toast

- Snack: Mixed nuts

- Lunch: Grilled shrimp salad with mixed greens and a vinaigrette dressing

- Snack: Sliced apple with almond butter

- Dinner: Baked cod with brown rice and roasted Brussels sprouts

Day 6:

- Breakfast: Smoothie with spinach, banana, and low-fat yogurt

- Snack: Sliced carrot sticks with hummus

- Lunch: Turkey and vegetable stir-fry with brown rice

- Snack: Low-fat cheese with whole-grain crackers

- Dinner: Baked tilapia with quinoa and steamed green beans

Day 7:

- Breakfast: Omelet with low-fat cheese, tomatoes, and bell peppers

- Snack: Strawberries with a dollop of whipped cream (unsweetened)

- Lunch: Chicken and vegetable kebabs with a side of couscous

- Snack: Baby tomatoes with balsamic vinegar

- Dinner: Pork tenderloin with mashed cauliflower and sautéed spinach

Certainly, here are the meal plans for Week 2 and Week 3 of a gestational diabetes diet:

Week 2:

Day 1:

- Breakfast: Scrambled eggs with spinach and whole-grain toast

- Snack: Greek yogurt with berries

- Lunch: Grilled chicken salad with mixed greens and vinaigrette dressing

- Snack: Baby carrots with hummus

- Dinner: Baked salmon with quinoa and steamed broccoli

Day 2:

- Breakfast: Oatmeal with sliced strawberries and a sprinkle of chopped nuts

- Snack: Cottage cheese with pineapple

- Lunch: Turkey and avocado wrap with a side salad

- Snack: Almonds and a small apple

- Dinner: Stir-fried tofu with mixed vegetables and brown rice

Day 3:

- Breakfast: Whole-grain pancakes with a small portion of blueberries

- Snack: Sliced cucumber with tzatziki sauce

- Lunch: Lentil soup with a side of mixed greens

- Snack: Sugar-free gelatin

- Dinner: Baked chicken breast with quinoa and roasted asparagus

Day 4:

- Breakfast: Greek yogurt parfait with low-sugar granola and raspberries

- Snack: Sliced bell peppers with guacamole

- Lunch: Spinach and feta stuffed chicken breast with a side of quinoa

- Snack: Celery sticks with peanut butter

- Dinner: Beef stir-fry with broccoli and cauliflower rice

Day 5:

- Breakfast: Scrambled egg whites with sautéed spinach and whole-grain toast

- Snack: Mixed nuts

- Lunch: Grilled shrimp salad with mixed greens and a vinaigrette dressing

- Snack: Sliced apple with almond butter

- Dinner: Baked cod with brown rice and roasted Brussels sprouts

Day 6:

- Breakfast: Smoothie with spinach, banana, and low-fat yogurt

- Snack: Sliced carrot sticks with hummus

- Lunch: Turkey and vegetable stir-fry with brown rice

- Snack: Low-fat cheese with whole-grain crackers

- Dinner: Baked tilapia with quinoa and steamed green beans

Day 7:

- Breakfast: Omelet with low-fat cheese, tomatoes, and bell peppers

- Snack: Strawberries with a dollop of whipped cream (unsweetened)

- Lunch: Chicken and vegetable kebabs with a side of couscous

- Snack: Baby tomatoes with balsamic vinegar

- Dinner: Pork tenderloin with mashed cauliflower and sautéed spinach

Week 3:

Repeat the Week 1 and 2 meal plan for Week 3 and 4 to maintain a consistent and balanced diet. Make adjustments based on your preferences and nutritional needs, and remember to monitor your blood sugar levels regularly.

If you enjoyed this book, please leave a positive review on the amazon site